Alkaline Diet

The Alkaline Meal Plan to Balance your pH, Reduce Body Acid, Lose Weight and Have Amazing Health

SECOND EDITION

By

Anne Wilson

Contents

INTRODUCTION 1

CHAPTER 1: What is the Alkaline Diet All About? 3

CHAPTER 2: Acidosis and the Body 9

CHAPTER 3: What are the Benefits of the Alkaline Diet? 15

CHAPTER 4: How to Get Started on the Alkaline Diet 23

CHAPTER 5: Top Foods to Alkalinize the Body 35

CHAPTER 6: Learn About Portion Control 45

CHAPTER 7: How Acids Affect the Glycemic Index 53

CHAPTER 8: Understanding Activity Levels and Energy
           Expenditures 57

CHAPTER 9: Specifics of Alkaline Cooking 59

CHAPTER 10: Diseases That Could Be Prevented—or
           Alleviated—by the Alkaline Diet 65

CHAPTER 11: FAQs 69

CHAPTER 12: Important Tips to Keep in Mind 75

CHAPTER 13: A Complete List of Alkalizing and
           Acidifying Foods 79

CONCLUSION 107

Introduction

I want to thank you and congratulate you for purchasing the book, *"Alkaline Diet: The Alkaline Meal Plan to Balance your pH, Reduce Body Acid, Lose Weight and Have Amazing Health"*.

This book contains proven steps and strategies on how to restore health by following the alkaline diet.

This diet plan is different from other popular diets. The aim is to restore the pH balance in the body. For what? First, most people have already accumulated too much acid in their body without their knowledge. Common foods and lifestyle promote acidity in the body, such as fast food, alcohol and lack of exercise. Acidity is not good for the body. It will promote health problems like cancer and diabetes. Find out more about the negative effects of acidity in the body. Furthermore, learn about how to reverse acidity by going on an alkaline diet. Learn more about the foods you can start eating today to restore pH balance. As a bonus, you also get a comprehensive list of foods that promote alkalinity and foods that produce acidity that you have to avoid.

Read more about the alkaline diet and how to start it today and soon, you will be on your way to reaping its many benefits, including better health and weight loss.

Thanks again for purchasing this book, I hope you enjoy it!

CHAPTER 1

What is the Alkaline Diet All About?

The Alkaline diet is also called the alkaline ash diet, acid ash diet, alkaline acid diet, or acid alkaline diet. This is actually a group of diets loosely related to each other. The main idea is that there are certain foods that directly affect the pH and acidity of the body's fluids, such as the blood and urine. This effect is believed to be therapeutic for certain health issues.

The Basics

The body has its own regulatory mechanism for balancing pH or its acid-base condition. The alkaline diet claims to help or boost this function. The traditional concept of the alkaline diet is to avoid eating poultry, meats, grains and cheese. The goal is to make the urine less acidic and more alkaline. This means increasing the urine's pH level. This is believed to help prevent the recurrence of UTIs (urinary tract infections) and discourage the formation of kidney stones (nephrolithiasis).

When eating foods, the body burns them to extract calories or energy. The extracted energy will then be used by the cells. If not, then some of these will be stored. This burning process is a slow and well-controlled one. So, when something gets burned, a residue is produced. It's like burning wood and ash is left behind. This ash is classified as either alkaline or acidic.

The Alkaline Diet was developed with the help of the US National Institute of Health as a means to lower blood pressure without the need for medication. Aside from being able to lower blood pressure, the Alkaline Diet has also proven to lower the risk of other diseases such as stroke, heart failure, diabetes, cancer, osteoporosis, and kidney stones. Not only will it work for you today, it's designed in such a way that it will have long term effects—so you can be sure that you'll be able to live a long and healthy life.

The Alkaline Diet is comprised of low-fat or non-fat dairy, fruits, vegetables, lean meats, whole grains, poultry, fish, beans, and nuts that are filled with various vitamins and minerals such as potassium, magnesium and calcium that your body certainly needs to develop and function. It is a diet that is high in fiber and low in fat so it would be easy for you to lose weight and lower your cholesterol levels and it also aims to reduce the amount of sodium that you consume so the systems of the body can be stabilized. This way, you can live your life the best way possible. Aside from eating the right kinds of food, it is also recommended that you lessen or quit smoking and exercise regularly so you can be sure that you'll be able to maintain your ideal weight and that a lot of diseases can be prevented.

If you choose to follow the ALKALINE diet, your systolic blood pressure will be able to drop by at least 7 to 12 points, which is a big help for your cholesterol levels to go down and make sure that you would not be suffering from any heart ailments or strokes anytime soon.

According to the diet, the acidity or alkalinity of the ash will have an effect on the body. Acidic ash will cause the body's fluids to become more acidic. Alkaline ash will cause the body's fluid pH to become more alkaline. Eating foods that produce neutral ash will have no effect on the body.

Acid ash is believed to increase the body's vulnerability to certain diseases. Alkaline ash is considered to have protective effects on the body. By eating more alkaline ash-producing foods, the body becomes "alkalinized" and health improves.

What composes the alkaline diet?

Recognized as a diet that most Hollywood celebrities love, the Alkaline Diet is said to help a person lose weight and also avoid certain diseases such as cancer, heart ailments, arthritis and Alzheimer's Disease. The said diet also keeps muscles and bones strong, making you a more active and reliable individual. It is also very beneficial when it comes to losing weight the right way in a short amount of time.

This is because the diet gets rid of some kinds of meat, processed foods, refined sugar and wheat that let your body produce the bad kind of acid which is not healthy for you. Meanwhile, if you eat the right kinds of food, then you can be sure that you'll be on the path to good health—and the Alkaline Diet has basically everything you need to be on the said path.

It is said that if you lessen the intake of acidic foods, then your body will not easily be susceptible to diseases and you'll be more active and energetic. It's also a way of cleaning up both your mind and body. In summation, the Alkaline Diet makes use of more meat and protein, and less carbohydrates. This is mainly because meat and protein were the staple foods of hunter-gatherers. However, one has to make sure that he gets to avoid trans fats, and omega-6 fats, because these wouldn't work well with the diet.

According to the diet, different kinds of foods have different effects in the body. Meats, grains, poultry, eggs, fish and cheese produce acid ash in the body. Vegetables and fruits, with the exception of plums, prunes and cranberries, produce alkaline ash. The designation of alkaline or acid ash depends on the effect of the food residue after combustion happens and not on the actual acidity of the food.

For example, citrus foods are known as acidic but in the alkaline diet, these are considered alkaline-producing foods because the residue has an alkalizing effect in the body.

The components of food determine whether the residue becomes acidic or alkaline. Components such as sulfur, phosphate and protein will leave acidic ash residue. Food components like calcium, potassium and magnesium will leave alkaline ash residue.

Food groups considered as acidic, neutral or alkaline include:

Acidic food group: eggs, dairy, fish, poultry, meats, alcohol and grains

Neutral food group: natural fats, sugars and starches

Alkaline food groups: nuts, vegetables, legumes and fruits

What is the body's pH and how is it regulated?

The body's pH refers to how acidic or alkaline the body fluids are. The pH range is:

Acidic: pH 0 to 6.99

Neutral: pH 7

Alkaline: pH 7.11 to 14

In the body, different fluids have different pH levels. It isn't uniform. For instance, the stomach is naturally acidic, even if there is no food. It becomes more acidic around mealtimes, contributing to the feelings of hunger. The acidity comes from the stomach acids, particularly HCl (hydrochloric acid). The normal stomach pH is 2 to 3.5, a highly acidic condition. Acidity is not always a bad thing in the body. The highly acidic environment of the stomach is necessary for digestion because it aids in breaking down tough food components.

The blood, on the other hand, needs a more alkaline environment. It normally has a pH of 7.35 to 7.45, which is in a slightly alkaline range. The blood pH has to be within the normal range at all times. If not, the cells will cease to function properly and a whole lot of serious health problems will develop. If the pH range is not within these values, there could be serious problems. If left untreated, it can turn fatal. However, problems with blood pH only happen as part of disease conditions. The food does not directly affect blood pH.

Thankfully, the body has an effective pH balancing mechanism called the acid-base homeostatic process. This involves the respiratory system and the metabolic system (gut). If the blood pH is acidic, the respirations speed up and the gut slows down to retain more base or alkaline compounds. If the blood pH becomes too alkaline, the respirations slow down and gut movement speeds up to lose more base or alkaline compounds. The urine also plays a part in balancing the blood pH.

What the foods affect is the pH of the urine. This is what the alkaline diet targets.

What makes food alkaline or acidic?

The pH of food in the alkaline diet depends on the pH of the residue once all its components are burned by the body. The most vital rule is that high alkaline foods are those that contain large amounts of alkaline minerals such as potassium, magnesium, sodium and calcium. However, even if a food does contain large amounts of these alkaline minerals, it may still be considered acidic if it also has any of the following:

- Sugar, especially added sugars and refined white sugar

- Fungi, such as mushrooms

- Yeast

- Fermented, such as soy sauce

- Processed, refined or microwaved

These standards explain why it is surprising to see certain acidic foods classified as alkaline in this diet plan. For example, fruits are considered healthy but are classified as acidifying because most of them have high sugar content. The sugar has an acidifying effect in the body. Another example is banana. It is an excellent source of the alkaline mineral potassium. However, it is classified as acidic food because it has about 25% sugar. Other fruits like lemon, lime, avocados and tomatoes are generally thought of as acidic foods, but in the alkaline diet, these fruits are classified as alkaline because these have low sugar.

Sugar is an important determinant in the alkaline diet. The blood can deviate from its normal pH range in the presence of too much sugar. This is a recipe for a double disaster. Too much sugar is a major factor in the development of diabetic condition and all its complications. The excess sugar load in the blood will acidify it and cause even more problems. This is a potent combination that can cause serious chronic health problems such as diabetes and cancer.

The longer this process continues, the more problems arise. These health problems will also become more serious and harder to treat, and all it takes is to simply adjust intake and concentrate on eating more alkaline foods.

CHAPTER 2

Acidosis and the Body

Acidic conditions in the body can come from various factors. It can be a result of emotional stress. It may also stem from toxin overload and/ or immune processes that reduce the amount of nutrients and oxygen reaching the cells. Of course, an acidic diet promotes acidic pH in the body. In response, the body will compensate by using its mineral stores to try to increase the pH towards the alkaline levels. If there aren't enough minerals available for the body to use, acid will build up within the cells and cause lots of health problems.

If the body is acidic, it will have decreased ability in absorbing minerals. That means less calcium, magnesium and phosphorus entering the bones, which will eventually lead to weaker bones. The muscles will also have decreased ability in absorbing potassium, calcium and magnesium. This can lead to weaker muscles, easy muscle fatigue, poor contraction and other similar muscle problems. If the muscles are not functioning well, several more problems can happen. The heart, which is all muscle, will not contract well and blood flow will be compromised. The gut, which is also composed of smooth muscles, will not contract and relax well. This can lead to poor digestion. There will be less nutrients available to the body, which will aggravate the problem.

On the cellular level, the cells' ability to repair itself will be compromised. This can lead to poor wound healing, decreased energy utilization, reduced ability of the body to protect itself from toxins and the proliferation of tumor cells. These are just a small portion of what can happen when the body is too acidic. The net effect of all these is increased likelihood for fatigue and risk for illnesses. Even the slightest dip in the body's pH level can turn fatal. For example, if the blood pH goes down to 6.9, coma and death can already occur.

Symptoms of Too Much Acid in the Body

Here is a list of common symptoms that indicate that the body is already too acidic. Presence of these symptoms should prompt you to make changes in your diet and choose to add more alkaline foods to daily meals to balance it.

Digestive issues, such as:

- Too much stomach acid
- Acid reflux
- Saliva is too acidic
- Ulcers
- Gastritis

Signs of Unhealthy Skin, Nails and Hair

- Dry skin
- Thinner nails that break easily
- Dull hair with split ends and easily falls out
- Cracks around the lip corners
- Pale face and skin all over the body
- Hives

Teeth and Mouth Issues

- Sensitive gums

- Loose teeth

- Teeth easily chip or crack

- Teeth become more sensitive to cold, hot or acidic foods

- Tooth nerve pain

- Mouth ulcers

- Frequent infections affecting the tonsils and throat

Head, Eyes, and Body in General

- Frequent headaches

- Leg cramps and spasms

- Body feels cold most of the time (low body temperature)

- Increased tendency to acquire infections

- Eyes tear easily

- Inflammation of the corneas and eyelids

- Conjunctivitis

- *Nerves and Emotions*

- Constant fatigue

- Low energy levels

- Anxiety or excessive nervousness

- Being continually depressed, often comes with loss of enthusiasm and joy for living, even for things that used to be enjoyable

Why are we getting acidic?

One of the main reasons why there is an acidic condition inside the body is the diet. A typical American diet consists of too many acid-producing foods. There are far too many animal products that produce acid ash in the body. These include dairy, eggs and meats. There are too few alkaline ash-producing foods like vegetables, and worse, there is too much intake of processed foods that also have acidifying effects in the body. Examples are foods made from white or refined flour, sugar and acidic drinks like sodas and coffee. Drugs are another reason. Chemical sweeteners like NutraSweet and Splenda are also contributing factors.

Emotions, too little exercise and stress contribute heavily to acid buildup in the body. Emotions, in particular, have twice the effect of food on the body. Exercise is necessary in the smooth flow of blood all over the body. Smooth blood flow helps in the proper delivery of oxygen and nutrients and in removing wastes.

What can be done?

To reduce the negative effects of acidic pH, it is advisable to change the diet to a more alkaline one. To maintain good health and optimum pH balance, put more focus on altering your diet. It is actually easier to make dietary and lifestyle changes to improve pH balance than to go down to the cellular level and treat pH imbalance.

Aside from concentrating in food, it is equally important to drink adequate amounts of water. Drink at least 3 to 4 liters of water, clean and unfiltered, each day. Again, not all types of water are the same. Distilled or purified water tends to be more on the acidic side. This is because distilled water has been stripped of the alkaline minerals.

The diet should be composed of 60% foods that form alkaline ash and the other 40% composed of acid-forming foods. This is the optimum for health maintenance. If there are already indications of poor health resulting from too much acidity, the diet should be at least 80% alkaline and 20% acid. It is still important to include acids in the diet to maintain balance. Otherwise, too much alkalinity will also create other types of problems.

CHAPTER 3

What are the Benefits of the Alkaline Diet?

The primary benefit of following the alkaline diet is that it restores or at least brings the body's pH from acidic to more alkaline. Too much acidity can produce lots of health problems and an alkaline diet can help prevent these.

Other benefits of following the alkaline diet go beyond the prevention of symptoms and problems related to too much acid. The alkaline environment helps tissues to function better.

Better energy

Cells must function well in order for the body to produce and use energy well. Acidity interferes with proper cellular processes and reduces energy levels. By going alkaline, the cells can function better. More energy will be produced and the other cells will have more to use for their own functions. This will result to higher energy levels.

Better gum and dental health

If the body is too acidic, the oral cavity is also acidic. Acidity will cause the dental enamel to erode, which will promote the formation of dental carries, plaques and cavities. This is also among the leading causes of bad breath. The acidic environment in the mouth promotes the overgrowth of bacteria. This will cause several oral health problems such as various gum diseases. This will also increase the risk for tooth decay. Most people notice improvement in their breath and overall dental health once they go on an alkaline diet.

Better immunity

When the various cells in the body are healthy, the immune system functions better. The integrity of the cells is great. Cellular integrity protects the cells from infections. The pathogens will find it difficult to enter and cause trouble. If the pH in the body is low (acidic), the cells will find it hard to keep their structures intact. This will allow toxins and pathogens to easily enter and cause more damage. These pathogens and toxins can easily get inside the cells and alter it. This will stimulate the development of health problems. Cancer, for instance, starts off this way. This is also a major reason why some people more frequently get colds and other infections compared to those who follow the alkaline diet.

Reduction in inflammation and pain

Magnesium is an important mineral in the body. It also has a vital role in maintaining the body's pH balance. If the body becomes acidic, the cells will release their magnesium stores to help in neutralizing the acidity. The more acidic the body, the more magnesium is required to counter its effects. This may be ideal but magnesium does not only function for acid neutralizing. The body has so many other uses for magnesium. Using a lot for acid neutralizing can seriously deplete the resources for the other tissues and cellular processes to use.

One of the major tissues affected is the joint. Low magnesium in the body is one of the factors that cause joint diseases and inflammatory conditions. Also, inflammation in the other tissues in the body is also attributed to low magnesium stores. Eating alkaline foods that are also rich in magnesium can replenish the resources and have more for the cells to use.

It strengthens the Neurons

When neurological processes are restored and protected, you get to protect yourself from Alzheimer's Disease and memory loss.

Degenerative diseases could also be prevented.

This happens because alkaline foods also contain L-Theanine, an amino acid that promotes better neurological health—and not a lot of food products are able to do this.

Better Weight Control

This is a culmination of all the positive effects of alkalinity in the body. The cells function better, so that energy is better distributed. Fats are used properly and the body has enough energy. This will reduce cravings and hunger cues. That means reduction in the frequency of hunger cues and better appetite control. Fats and energy are also burned much better, reducing the risk of accumulating more fats that contribute to weight gain.

Preventing Stomach Upset

Thermogenesis, the term given to fat to energy conversion, is increased by at least 8 to 10 % when someone uses alkaline foods in his daily diet. This not only burns fat, but also regulates the digestive process.

Alkaline foods also reduce intestinal gas, and could also prevent certain diseases from happening, such as ulcers, ulcerative colitis, and Chron's Disease.

Slower Aging Process

The aging process is driven by the damage to cells. When cells easily degrade and repair is slow, the aging process is accelerated. If the cells are able to repair damage efficiently and at a faster rate, the aging process slows down. In an acidic environment, the cells get easily damaged and at a much faster rate. Repair is slowed in acidic pH. In an alkaline environment, cells do not get as much damage and when any injury gets repaired sooner.

Also, the aging process is accelerated due to oxidative stress. This is caused by the accumulation of free radicals and toxins that eat away at the cells. Acidic pH in the body supports oxidative stress. Alkaline pH helps in reducing the toxin load and oxidative stress. These promote younger-looking, healthier cells that give a younger appearance.

Perfect for Athletes

This is mainly because they know that if they eat too much fat, their bodies would suffer, and their hearts would grow weaker—and that's never a good thing because they live such active lives. Even superstars such as LeBron James have actually pledged allegiance to the low carb diet—so why won't you?

More so, when you adhere to these diets, it would be easy for your body to turn nutrients into ketogenic energy. When you have ketones in your system, you get to perk yourself up, and you get to have enough energy to get through the day—and help you out with whatever it is that you have to do!

Plus, when it comes to weight loss, you really cannot expect that you'd lose weigh if you keep on eating too much fats and carbohydrates. It's just not right, and won't work well with what you have in mind. Since regular exercise is said to work best with the Alkaline Diets, you can keep in mind that you could make it a part of your life—so you could be sure that the diet would really work.

Avoiding Chronic Inflammation

Chronic inflammation is the reason why so many diseases happen. These diseases include Type 2 Diabetes, Heart Problems, and Cancer. This so happens because grains are—you guessed it—inflammatory. While you may not see the effects right away, in time, you'd notice how your body would disintegrate, and how you'd feel like you're no longer in shape, and that your health is on the downlow. When you keep on eating grains, you're just fueling up the problem instead of working on ways to solve it.

Staying away from Auto-Immune Diseases

Take a look at it this way: Gliadin, also known as the worst kind of gluten, is actually responsible for affecting the pancreas, thyroids, and the entire immune system by means of releasing antibodies that aren't meant to get out yet. When these antibodies go out, auto-immune diseases come into play and one may be afflicted with diseases such as Hashimoto's Disease, type 1 diabetes, and hypothyroidism, among others.

Incidentally, research has it that Alzheimer's Disease is often triggered by high-grain diets. It releasers blockers in the brain that could break mental processes down, and therefore lead to the deterioration of the brain.

Develop a Healthy Gut

Doctors believe that the state of your gut could affect the state of your brain. After all, when you're hungry, you tend to make decisions that are not well thought out.

As you can see, your gut is in charge of a lot of things in your body—which you often fail to see in your daily life. These things include the way you utilize fat and carbohydrates; nutrient absorption; being satiated; vitamin and neurotransmitter production; inflammation; detoxification, and immunity against diseases, amongst others.

This is also because of the vagus nerve, found in the gut, which is the longest of the 12 cranial nerves. This is the main channel between your digestive system, and your nerve cells that send signals to the brain.

In short, it would be wrong for you not to take care of your gut because it would be like a way of putting your own health in danger. Why?

Well, because if the given processes above does not work right, you might be afflicted with certain medical conditions, such as dementia, diabetes, allergies, cancer, ADHD, asthma, and other chronic health problems.

Not only that, the clarity of your thoughts, and the way you feel are also affected. When you don't eat what's right for you, you might be afflicted with anxiety, depression, or other problems that won't make life easy for you.

When your gut is healthy, your brain gets to make more serotonin—the hormone that keeps you happy, and keeps your sanity in check—one that not even the best anti-depressants could give out too much, and this is why you have to make sure that you start eating right.

Avoid Vitamin-D Deficiency

Even if you consume Vitamin D, it actually depletes inside the body pretty fast, and acid makes depletion even faster. More so, WGA, or Wheat Germ Agglutinin also causes bacterial growth that kills Vitamin D, and damages the gut—and could do much worse to your body in the future.

Dehydration Will Be Prevented

Unlike coffee and soda, alkaline food makes an amazing drink because it keeps the body hydrated, and makes sure that dehydration is prevented. Alkaline food has moisture, as mentioned in an earlier chapter, which means that it actually has water, unlike other flavored or carbonated drinks.

You're on the Road to Feeling So Much Better

It sounds cheesy, sure, but the thing is when you adhere to these diet combination, it's like you're giving yourself the chance to feel good again.

These days, people go through a lot of things. Their lives—possibly yours, too—could turn nasty in just a second, and it would be even harder if they don't take care of their health. So, as early as now, you should consider this book a chance for you to reverse your health—for the better, of course!

Top Health Benefits from a well-balanced pH in the body

- Skin has better elasticity and looks more radiant and youthful

- Sleep is deeper and more restful

- Abundant physical energy

- Reduced frequency of suffering from colds, flu viruses and headaches

- Improved digestion

- Reduced symptoms of arthritis

- Reduction of overgrowth of yeast (*Candida* infection)

- Reduced risk for osteoporosis

- Improvement of mental acuity and better mental alertness

- Safe, healthy, legal natural high from better hormonal and neurotransmitter levels

CHAPTER 4

How to Get Started on the Alkaline Diet

To start the alkaline diet, prepare yourself for a lifetime of dietary changes. It is not a short-term, one-time only diet like most people associate with the term "diet". It is a long-term decision. Knowing the right foods that produce the desired healthy benefits will greatly help you succeed in making your body more alkaline.

Change how you view food

The very first step is to change the way you look at and treat food itself. Take this time to evaluate yourself. Is food merely for sustenance? Is it merely a source of calories? Or is it a source of energy and materials that the body can use to be healthy?

Food should not just be a source of energy. If this is your view, you are most likely to be not too concerned on quality. Rather, it's more on quantity. The right thinking should be on the quality of food. The alkaline diet teaches you to be more aware of the things you eat and how it ultimately affects the balance in your body. What are the ingredients in food? Does it supply the body's nutritional requirements? Does it contain potentially harmful components? What is the body's reaction to the various components of food?

Also, never think that diets are just about counting calories. What's important is that you aid your diet with exercise. Anyway, when you eat well regularly, you already get to lose around 500 calories—so there's really no need to starve yourself!

Get a list of the different types of foods and how they affect the body. A comprehensive list is available at the end of this book. Use this list as a guide on what to include in meals, what to limit and what to avoid.

Drink lots of pure, clean water

Water is vital for normal functioning of the various tissues. In fact, about 70% of the body is composed of water. It is used as a medium for various cellular processes. It is also used to dilute salts, toxins and other substances to keep them under control. Water is used as a medium for excreting wastes and toxins. It is crucial to replenish water stores in the body because it can be easily depleted through sweat, tears, urine, feces, etc.

As the human body is made up of 75% water, it comes as no surprise that a person needs to be able to sustain that amount. If a person loses water in his system, he will be dehydrated and it would be hard to live a happy and healthy life. Because of this, it's important to understand how vital water is for you and how much of it you need per day. Water also aids in weight loss. Because it has no preservatives and is not carbonated, it doesn't add any calories or carbohydrates to your body, which is essential for people who want to lose weight.

Surprisingly, water nowadays is acidic. Try to test various commercial bottled water brands and you'll see they are acidic. The usual pH range would be as acidic as pH 4 to 6. Drinking lots of water is good, but not if it's acidic. It will only add more acidity inside the body. Choose clean, pure water. If possible, get spring water, with all the natural dissolved minerals in it. Distilled water in bottles is already stripped off of all the dissolved substances that are beneficial to the body.

Sometimes, the weather gets too hot that a person may feel dehydrated. To prevent being sick or experiencing heat stroke because of extremely hot weather, it's important that a person drinks 13 to 15 cups of water per day or that he eats fruits that are loaded with fluids, too. Aside from water, a person with fever or diarrhea may also have to take oral supplements or sports drinks to replenish the loss of water in his system. You can also try fruits such as watermelons or pears—they're pretty much filled with water and that's why they are good for you.

Also, if you are fond of working out or of any activity that makes you sweat then you certainly need to drink a lot of water to make up for what you have lost. You need to add 1 to 3 more cups to your usual intake.

Aside from water, you could also drink the following:

- **Coconut Water.** Coconut Water is dubbed as nature's own sports drink that has a thermogenic effect and helps make sure that the gut is strong and safe.

- **Juice.** Not the processed kind, though. Try to make your own green juices (with vegetables as base), and mix and match ingredients. It's actually fun, and you'd also help yourself gain a lot of nutrients by doing so, too. Try using the following: *cucumber, celery, beet, carrot, ginger, parsley, spinach, and cabbage.* Then add either of the following: *berries, watermelon, aloe vera, goji berry, acai berry, etc.*

- **Shakes and Smoothies.** Shakes and smoothies are fine, as long as you made them yourself, and they do not contain additives.

- **Tea.** Herbal teas, as you may know by now, are important parts of your diet. Make sure you do not add sugar or milk, though. 3 to 5 cups per day is already good.

The lack of dissolved substances makes distilled water more acidic than regular, clean water. Instead of getting distilled water, choose filtered water. It still retains some of the valuable dissolved materials and is less acidic.

Make various meals out of cruciferous vegetables

Here's the thing: the more alkaline foods you eat, the more you lose weight. When you chew alkaline foods, it automatically means that you are already burning and digesting your food—and of course, it's only natural that you get to chew these vegetables, especially if you eat them instead of your usual snacks or fatty foods, in general. If you want to eat your snacks, you need to have the mindset of eating a whole bunch of cruciferous vegetables first—so later, you'd only eat a small amount of the snacks.

Cruciferous vegetables come from the Cruciferae Family. These are vegetables that are generally cultivated for food production. Interestingly, the name also originated from "Cruciferae", which in early Latin literally means "cross-bearing", an allusion to the shape of the flowers that seem to resemble crosses. Prime examples of cruciferous vegetables include: *Brussels sprouts, bok choy, garden cress, broccoli, cabbage,* and *cauliflower.*

These vegetables are known to be essential parts of the Negative Calorie Diet because they are high in cellulose, water, and Vitamin C, together with essential phytochemicals and nutrients that the body needs.

Most cruciferous vegetables also contain glucosinulates that are said to prevent cancer, drive toxins away from the body, and could suit the taste of many—and that's why they are used in most plant-based recipes!

You see, your overall calorie intake will ultimately be reduced when you eat alkaline foods instead of high-calorie ones—and if you exercise as you do so, you'd really see substantial amount of weight loss.

Once you start the diet, you'd really notice that you are losing weight. Over time, though, you might feel a lack of energy—but then you'd also realize that as your metabolism slows down, it would then work to provide you with more energy—which will then be used by your body as fuel to live!

What you should keep in mind, though, is that you have to eat at least every 2 to 3 hours—so you could sustain the energy that your body needs, and you also have to take note that you cannot eat sugar or honey—and other sugar replacements, with the exception of Stevia. It's also important not to use any artificial dressings because more often than not, they contain sugar. For dressings, you could use garlic or Dijon mustard mixed with yogurt and your choice of herbs.

Evaluate food on hand

Most of the time, there isn't any real need to throw everything that's already in the fridge or pantry and buy new kinds of food. There are no specialized food requirements for the alkaline diet. It's actually a simple type of diet, utilizing the common everyday food items. Check whatever is on hand and compare them to the list. If there are acidic foods, which is highly probable there will be, there's no need to throw them out. A great thing about the alkaline diet is that foods can be mixed to get a healthier dish.

Mix acidic foods with alkaline foods to balance out the acidity. For instance, herbs are a great way of balancing the pH of meals. Mix ginger with beef to even out the pH. Add curry spices to chicken to reduce its acid-forming effect. Not only do herbs balance the pH, these are also excellent at adding more flavor to meals. Another example of mixing foods to balance the pH is by wrapping bacon around asparagus sticks and grill or steam it. Drizzle healthy alkalizing oils over acidic foods to improve the pH. The omega-3 fats from these oils will help create a more alkaline environment in the body. Be creative. There is no need for specialized food items.

It would also help you to be on the lookout for macronutrients, also known as macros. These measure your daily intake of carbohydrates, protein, and fats. The amount that you should take might be different from everybody else's, so you do have to know exactly where you stand. For this, you have to understand that it would be important to know your measurements, starting with the size of your waist. To know the accurate size of your waist, go get a tape measure. Then, find the widest point around your belly button, and measure from there—and not from where you have placed your belt at. Then, go ahead and learn what your real weight is by weighing yourself first thing in the morning—without any clothes on.

Once you know that, you have to enter your body weight in lbs and in kilograms, and you also have to know what your body fat percentage is. If you have no idea what you body fat percentage is, you could keep the following in mind:

- **10-14%.** This is usually called the beach body look. Muscles and fat may be separated, but you may not see it in every muscle group. There might also be veins on the arms and legs.

- **5-9%.** This means that there's a lot of vascularity in the muscles—think body builders, or athletes, especially those who wrestle or play football, boxing even. The abs would also be well-defined—which means body fat is pretty low.

- **15-19%.** With these percentages, you could expect that there is less vascularity and that muscles are also not that defined anymore. You could see a great separation between them—except for the arms.

- **20-24%.** This is another common type of body fat percentage. The muscle and fat separation is almost non-existent, and the muscle groups are also not strained or vascular—making them easier on the eyes. Aim for this one.

- **25-29%.** This is already considered obese, at least, for men. This is because it's obvious how the stomach is already round, and that the waist has also increased or has widened. Neck fat may also be there, but veins and muscles may not be around.

- **30-34%.** This means that the hips are smaller than the body and waist—too much fat is visible.

This way, you would know the right portions that can help you—which you'll learn more about in Chapter 6.

Learn to listen to "hunger cues"

Pay attention to how you feel and if you know you're already hungry, go ahead and eat something, but try to scale it out. For example, ask yourself if you really are hungry in a span of 1 to 10, 10 being the highest. By questioning yourself, you'd know if you actually should eat already, but again, do not starve yourself at all.

Start slowly

To avoid getting overwhelmed with all the changes in following the alkaline diet, start slowly. Incorporate 2 to 3 alkaline meals per week. There is no need to totally change your entire week's menu just to follow this diet plan. You can start slowly as you gradually replace whatever acidic foods you have at present with more alkaline ones. Slowly add more alkaline recipes until you have at least 10 to 20 different alkaline meals per week. These meals should be tasty, so you can still enjoy the foods you want. Again, the key is to balance acidic with alkaline foods. This way, you can also curb any cravings that will come as you make the transition to a full alkaline diet.

How can you make better food choices to improve pH?

Food choices are the cornerstone to improving and balancing pH levels of the body. Everything ultimately depends on what foods were chosen to become part of each and every meal, including snacks. Making the right choice every time is not always easy. To get through the tougher times, live by these guidelines:

- Choose white meat over red meats. Healthier meat alternatives also include meat substitutes and seafood.

- Choose wild rice or yeast-free bread instead of fries or rolls.

- Choose almond milk instead of cow's milk.

- Choose sparkling water instead of alcoholic beverages.

- Choose vegetables as main dishes instead of starches or meats.

- Choose to fill the plate first with plant foods like vegetables, grains and fruits so that there is little space left for acid-forming food items.

- Choose vegetables with dips or fresh grilled fruit instead of prepackaged or processed snacks.

- Choose to use cold-pressed olive oil for cooking instead of butter or saturated fats.

- Choose to have dressings, sauces and condiments on the side instead of having them already mixed into the food when eating out or ordering take-out.

- Choose to exercise every day, like walking for at least 30 minutes instead of watching a 30-minute TV show.

- Choose to reduce the stress levels by performing yoga, meditation and other similar relaxation techniques.

How to monitor the pH level of the body?

The simplest and easiest method of monitoring acidity in the body is by checking the urine pH. This is not a requirement to be successful but it immensely helps in checking how well the body responds to the diet. Urine pH monitoring can help in tailoring the diet according to your body's needs. Some people can restore alkalinity by just adding more alkalizing vegetables. Some may need to make huge cut-backs in their meat consumption. Responses are different among individuals and the change is a personal thing. To make the alkaline diet more suitable for your needs, monitor urine pH levels to evaluate your body's responses.

Testing is done every day. Early morning urine is the best sample that can give more reliable results compared to random urine sampling throughout the day. There are ready to use test strips available in pharmacies that you can use to test urine pH levels at the comfort of your home. These test strips can give reliable pH readings without having to take the urine sample to laboratories or medical clinics.

To use the urine pH test strip:

- Remove the test strip from the package. If the test kit comes in a roll, carefully tear off a 3-inch piece.

- Sit down on the toilet bowl and start to urinate. Catch the midstream urine for the test sample. The first few ml of urine (the first 2 seconds worth of urine) is most acidic than the rest and is not the most reliable sample. Readings will give a false positive result. This means getting a very acidic urine pH that's not an actual representation of the entire urine pH. The higher acidity readings is a result of sitting and getting more concentrated in the urinary bladder compared to the rest of the urine.

- Once in midstream, take the urine test strip and place it directly under the stream of urine. Hold it there until the strip is thoroughly moistened.

- Take the test strip then compare it immediately to the chart that comes with the test kit. Match the color of the moistened test strip with the keyed color chart printed on the side of test bottle or of the packaging.

- The number that best matches the color of the test strip will be the urine sample's pH level.

- Record the result. Use this for future reference.

- Discard used test strip properly. These strips are not reusable.

- Testing the urine pH can be done as often as desired. However, once per day is enough to gauge the body's pH level for that day.

Be Consistent

Don't try to lose weight today and then go ahead with your bad eating habits again next week. What's important here, as well as in any kind of diet, is consistency. You have to make sure that you are committed to it and that you don't give in to temptation. For this, it would be nice to keep a food journal and make sure to fill it up with information regarding what you just ate, and add some healthy recipes—those you'll find in this book, too!

How to make correct exchanges from common acidic foods to more alkaline choices?

To make meal more alkaline, reduce the amount and frequency of acidic foods. There are alkaline substitutes available for common food items that you can use to enjoy tasty meals, beverages and snacks while balancing the body's pH.

Acidic Food	Substitute with
Butter	Clarified butter; cold-pressed olive oil
Flour	Almond flour or skinless almonds finely crushed
White rice	Basmati or wild rice
White potatoes	Sweet potatoes
Yeast breads	Sprouted grains
Yeast	Lemon juice and baking soda
Soda	Sparkling water
Coffee	Herbal tea
Creamer	Almond milk
Canned fruits	Frozen fruits, no additives
Gelatin (made from meat or animal parts like knuckles)	Agar-agar (made from seaweeds)
Condiments	Fresh spices and herbs
Sugar	Clover honey, Stevia
Peanuts	Chestnuts, almonds
Navy beans	Lentils
Whole eggs	Egg whites
Red meats	Firm tofu, poultry

CHAPTER 5

Top Foods to Alkalinize the Body

To get started on the alkaline diet, here are the top alkaline ash-producing foods that you can start to include in your diet right now:

Almond, Almond Milk

Almonds, in any type of diet or list, are consistently at the top of the healthiest foods to include. It's also a top alkaline food and is very versatile. You can toast it and add it to salads, smoothies or baked products. You can use it for almond-crusted meats, fish or poultry to balance the pH of a dish. Almonds are also perfect as simple, hassle-free snacks. Just limit the consumption to not more than a handful a day.

Aside from its alkaline effect, almonds also promote other health benefits. These are linked to better lean muscle gain, aids in fat loss (resulting in healthier weight loss), and helps in decreasing levels of cholesterol in the body.

Almond milk is a great alternative to dairy milk. This is healthier and less likely to cause any digestive concerns that regular dairy milk does in sensitive people. It is a great alternative for those who are struggling with weight issues and allergic or intolerance conditions. Just use it in place of milk, such as in smoothies.

Nutritional profile (per 100 grams):

Calcium content: 27%

Protein content: 44%

Iron content: 25%

Artichokes

These are commonly added to salads or in dips, but this humble artichoke can be used as a main ingredient instead of just an addition. Its alkalizing effect helps in raising the pH in the body and in promoting better health. Aside from that, artichokes contain lots of antioxidants that aid in detoxifying the liver and in improving the digestive process.

Artichokes are often seen on top of salads, or used in a dip, but there are a number of reasons why you can bring them to the forefront of your diet. One of those reasons is their alkalinity, helping to raise your body's pH levels. They're also full of antioxidants, help to purify the liver, and aid in digestion.

Use artichokes more often and in larger amounts. For example, grilled artichokes make great pairings with meats to balance the pH.

Nutritional profile (per 100 grams):

Vitamin K: 12%

Vitamin C: 20%

Folates: 17%

Arugula

Calcium is usually abundant in dairy foods, but there are other rich, non-dairy sources as well such as arugula. This is another great leafy green worth knowing and adding to daily meals. This leafy green is more commonly added to detoxifying diet plans. It is one of the top alkaline foods to try. Arugula is abundant in Vitamin A and has impressive calcium content.

Aside from being low in calories, it's also low in cholesterol and fat—which most health-conscious people don't want in their diets, too. On the other hand, it is high in potassium, Vitamins C, K, and A, fiber, and other important nutrients. Arugula is also filled with antioxidants that drive toxins away—and kills free radicals that damage the body.

Nutritional profile (per 100 grams):

Calcium: 16%

Iron: 8%

Vitamin A: 47%

Asparagus

This is an effective food when it comes to promoting alkalinity in the body. This is among the top ranked foods in the alkaline diet, but aside from alkalizing the body, arugula brings so much more. It is known as one of the most traditional detoxifying foods because it's able to act as a diuretic that drives toxins away and speeds up metabolism in the body. It also contains important vitamins and minerals, such as protein, copper, iron, folate, and Vitamins B6, K, E, C, and A, among others.

It is chock full of antioxidants and nutrients. It also has lots of detoxifying properties that promote better health. This crunchy green is also reported to have effective anti-aging effects.

Nutritional profile (per 100 grams):

Vitamin C: 9%

Vitamin A: 15%

Iron: 12%

Avocado & Avocado Oil

Avocado is rich in healthy fats that promote various health benefits. This is also among the top alkaline foods that you should include in daily meals. There are so many ways to add avocados. Try them as part of power-packed smoothies, as sweet addition to salads, as desserts on their own or as dip (guacamole). Avocados are also packed with Vitamin K that promotes alkalinity and other health benefits.

Avocado oil is another powerful alkalizing food. It makes a great substitute to unhealthy acidic oils.

Nutritional profile (per 100 grams):

Vitamin A: 3%

Fiber: 27%

Vitamin C: 17%

Basil

Not all people realize that spices and herbs have notable effects in their bodies. These are more than just aromatics and flavorings. These also influence the acidity or alkalinity of the body. Basil is one of the best herbs that promote alkalinity. Aside from this, basil contains a good amount of flavonoids that promote health and healing.

Nutritional profile (per 100 grams):

Vitamin A: 175%

Calcium: 18%

Vitamin K: 345%

Buckwheat

This is a rising star among the health food circle. It does not contain wheat, even if the name has the word "wheat" in it. This is fast becoming a widely used healthier alternative to wheat. Noodles made of buckwheat have very similar texture to those made of wheat. This makes it a great alternative to wheat pasta, allowing people to enjoy pasta dishes without the negative effects from wheat.

Buckwheat also lowers the acidity in the body, so people do not have to worry about acidity. Aside from its alkaline effects, buckwheat is also a great source of healthy proteins, with a good amount of iron as well. There are so any recipes to try using buckwheat so start adding this to daily meals.

Nutritional profile (per 100 grams):

Protein: 13.3 grams

Calcium: 2%

Iron: 12%

Carrot

These are great vegetables for improved eye health. It also has great alkalizing effects in the body. These are tasty whether raw or cooked. Carrots are rich in carotenoids, vitamins, potassium and fiber.

Nutritional profile (per 100 grams):

Vitamin A: 336%

Calcium: 3%

Vitamin C: 10%

Cauliflower

This belongs to the same vegetable family as Brussels sprouts and broccoli. These are all cruciferous vegetables. These share the same nutritional characteristics and all promote alkaline environments in the body. Cauliflower is a great source of folate. It's also filled with lots of Vitamin C and phytonutrients that help you lose weight, and prevent the formation of cancer. It's also a good rice substitute, and is one of the most important superfoods around.

Cauliflower, in particular, has a good amount of fiber. This is also a great source of vitamin C, comparable to the amounts found in fruits. Cauliflower is best eaten raw to retain most of its alkaline-promoting compounds.

Nutritional profile (per 100 grams):

Vitamin C: 77%

Iron: 2%

Calcium: 2%

Celery

Some people may not be keen on the taste of raw celery sticks but its nutritional offers are so much worth it. It is a highly alkaline food that can promote balance in the body's pH levels. Celery contains low amounts of calories but it is very filling. This is perfect for those who want to promote alkalinity in the body and those who are trying to lose weight. Munch on fresh celery sticks or add them to smoothies for some more spiciness.

Nutritional profile (per 100 grams):

Vitamin A: 4%

Calcium: 2%

Vitamin C: 2%

Other Alkalizing Foods

Apart from these top alkalizing foods, here are a few more items to add to improve the pH balance in the body.

Alkalizing Protein

Meats and other animal protein sources are top acidifying foods, but this does not mean that you should eliminate protein from your diet. Protein is important in promoting health and wellness. There are protein sources that have alkalizing effect in the body, so make sure to add these:

- Chestnuts
- Almonds
- Millet
- Tofu (fermented)
- Tempeh (fermented)
- Whey Protein Powder

Alkalizing Sweeteners

Sugar is an acidifying food ingredient. Natural sugars in food have alkalizing effect but added ones like added refined sugars will acidify the body. Artificial sweeteners used in place of refined white sugar are also acidifying. One safe, alkalizing artificial sweetener is Stevia.

Alkalizing Spices & Seasonings

Seasonings and spices are simple and easy ways to turn acidic meals to more alkaline.

- Herbs (all)
- Cinnamon
- Chili Pepper
- Curry

- Ginger

- Miso

- Sea Salt

- Mustard

- Tamari

Other Alkalizing Foods

A few more other foods that can help in reversing acidity and restoring pH balance in the body include:

- Alkaline Antioxidant Water

- Mineral Water

- Bee Pollen

- Apple Cider Vinegar

- Green Juices

- Fresh Fruit Juice

- Molasses, blackstrap

- Soured Dairy Products

- Probiotic Cultures

- Veggie Juices

- Lecithin Granules

Alkalizing Minerals

Minerals in food and supplements can also help in alkalizing the body. The best ones are:

- Sodium: pH 14

- Potassium: pH 14

- Cesium: pH 14

- Calcium: pH 12

- Magnesium: pH 9

CHAPTER 6

Learn About Portion Control

Another thing that you have to understand about the Alkaline Diet is that it is essential for you to choose proper portions. When you portion your food, it becomes easier for you to make sense of what you're eating—and because of that, you can get more of the nutrients that you need, too.

Start with meat...and all kinds of protein

So, what should make up your portions, then? First, you can start with Protein, which definitely includes turkey or chicken breasts, salmon, tuna, halibut, pork loin or pork chops, non-fat mozzarella cheese, tofu, beans, lean beef, veal, soy milk, yogurt, nuts and seeds, eggs, and egg whites. Protein is one of the body's essential nutrients because it is very beneficial. It can repair and replace tissues, hair, blood, nails and even muscles and a person needs to sustain the amount of protein in his system so that he would not easily be susceptible to diseases. For athletes, protein is important because it builds muscles instead of fat and keeps them sturdy and on their feet. Body-builders rely on Protein a lot, too. Protein is also considered as the building blocks of tissue, which means that it can also be considered as one of life's building blocks. Without it, a person will feel unhealthy and would not be able to function well.

The recommended amount of Protein always depends on your age, sex, weight and level of activity. Around 50 to 175 grams per day is generally good. This also means that you can eat at least 5 to 6 ounces of protein-rich food each day. Men also need more Protein than women. If a woman eats 6 ounces of Protein each day, a man has to eat 7 to 8. Adults also need more Protein than children and so do bodybuilders. A bodybuilder has to eat 6 to 9 grams of protein per every pound of his weight. Other active adults have to eat 4 to 5 grams of protein each day, too.

Lots of vegetables

This should make up at least ¾ of your plate. Most vegetables have low acid content. Males need around 2 to 3 cups of vegetables daily while women need 2 to 2 ½ cups. The same level goes for fruits. However, the amount may change depending on the kind of activity you do, your gender and also your age. Take note that again, men need more vegetables than women and that if they are extremely active or if they do 60 or more minutes of physical activity daily, they would need 4 to 5 cups of vegetables and around 3 to 4 cups of fruits. Kids need around 1 to 3 cups of vegetables and 2 to 3 cups of fruits daily.

Vegetables help reduce the risk of heart diseases such as heart attacks and stroke and can also protect the body against certain types of cancer. Vitamin C aids against inflammation and helps wounds heal fast. Plus, it also protects the body against several types of infections. Vegetables are also great sources of essential nutrients such as Vitamin C, Vitamin A, Folate and Dietary Fiber. Fiber not only aids in weight loss but also cleans the systems of the body and rids it of toxins. Aside from that, it's also important in regulating bowel movement. When this happens, it will be easy for you to digest food and be able to get the nutrients you need from the foods you eat. Fiber heightens the body's metabolic levels, too.

As some vegetables are high in potassium, it means that they can lower your blood pressure, decrease the level of bone loss and can also help in lowering blood pressure, as well. Some vegetables that are rich in potassium include potatoes, sweet potatoes, lima beans, beet greens, lentils, soy beans, tomatoes, tomato products and kidney beans, as well. Vegetables are rich in fiber so they can prevent obesity and Type

II Diabetes and can definitely aid in making you lose weight fast.

Vegetables also keep the skin healthy and radiant, and vegetables that are rich in folate are great for pregnant and lactating women. These vegetables give them a chance to produce healthier kinds of milk. Aside from this, Folate also provides the body with healthy red blood cells which means that you will not be easily susceptible to diseases and that you can absorb other nutrients easily. Folate also protects the body against certain diseases such as spina bifida, tube defects and ancephaly that are easily gotten when the baby is still inside the mother's womb. As you can see, eating vegetables can help protect the baby and make sure that he gets out well and healthy.

To make portion control easier, you can make use of the following vegetables:

- **Lettuce.** Aside from extremely low amount of acid, what you can expect about lettuce is that no matter how much you eat of it, it still won't make you gain a lot of weight. Lettuce that contain the most nutrients are red leaf, purple, or dark green.

- **Brussels Sprouts**. What's great about Brussels sprouts is that they're loaded with fiber and phytonutrients that make you lose weight and that prevent cancer. Sure, you may not like them at first, but when cooked right, they actually taste amazing.

- **Beets**. What's amazing about beets is that although they are sweet, they actually do not contain sugar and they are also filled with fiber, antioxidants, potassium, folate, and iron!

- **Mushrooms.** Mushrooms are not just the favorite pizza toppings of some, they're also quite amazing because they could boost and protect the immune system as they contain fiber, B Vitamins, potassium, and loads of antioxidants! The best variants include Portobello, Shitake, and White, amongst others.

- **Turnips.** Turnips promise low glycemic index, which means you'll also be protected from diabetes, and is also one of the best sources of Vitamin C.

- **Spinach.** Another miraculous vegetable, spinach is quite flavorful. It contains Vitamin K, Folic Acid, iron, beta-carotene, and phytonutrients that help you lose weight and protect you against loads of diseases. It also prevents macular degeneration.

- **Zucchini.** Another favorite, zucchini is sometimes known as the "miracle squash" because it allows you to feel satiated— without filling you up with calories. It's also filled with Vitamin A!

- **Garlic.** Garlic is amazing because it strengthens the immune system and helps fight colds, together with most urinary infections. It has lots of antimicrobial and antiviral properties!

- **Kale.** One of those vegetables that are part of many diet regimens these days, Kale is a great superfood that prevents breast cancer and is also filled with lots of phytonutrients. Aside from that, it's also one of the best sources of manganese, folic acid, and most vitamins, as well.

- **Carrots.** They are so low in cholesterol and fat, which makes them a perfect part of this diet. They're also rich in beta-carotene and Vitamin A—essential nutrients that the body needs.

- **Celery.** What's great about celery is that it's filled with cellulose and it's considered a high volume food—which means that even if you eat a lot, you won't get fat. It's perfect for those who are trying to have healthy pregnancies, and is also filled with folate, vitamin C, and vitamin A, among others.

- **Fennel.** This prevents winter coughs, boosts your immune system, and is filled with lots of vitamins and minerals, as well.

- **Radishes.** They aid in digestion because they contain lots of sulfur compounds, antioxidants, and folic acid, and has twice the amount of calcium that leafy vegetables have.

- **Pumpkins**. Pumpkins have many antioxidants, beta-carotene, and essential vitamins. It's also so easy to add to a lot of dishes, so it's a great part of any diet! It lowers blood pressure, as well.

Add some carbohydrates

Next, you also have to realize that carbohydrates are not actually *that* bad. In fact, you need a good amount of them to help you ease through life, and make sure your weight would not fluctuate since you are trying to get rid of acidic foods. Carbohydrates are important to your body when taken in the right amount. Carbohydrates are essential because they boost your mood and increase the amounts of "happy hormones" in your body; they keep the memory sharp; they are good for your heart and have the right amount of soluble fiber that you need. Eating 5 to 10 grams of carbohydrates daily can lessen the amount of cholesterol in your system by at least 5 percent, and; they help control the amount of fat in your body, making sure that fat gets turned into glucose—which your body could then use as "energy" or fuel to live.

For this, you can try quinoa, whole wheat pizza, barley, bulgur, or popcorn. Basically, the mount of carbohydrates that you need depends on your lifestyle. For example, people who are lean and who regularly work out needs just 100 to 150 grams of carbohydrates per day. This means that they can eat all the vegetables they want together with some fruits and healthy starches such as potatoes, oats and rice.

If someone wants to lose weight but still cannot give up carbohydrates, he is allowed to eat 5o to 100 grams of carbohydrates per day. This means that he has to eat plenty of vegetables, around 2 to 3 pieces of fruits and a minimal amount of starchy carbohydrates. For those who want to boost their metabolism or want to lose weight fast but still in the natural manner, they are supposed to eat 20 to 50 grams of fat each day. They have to eat plenty of vegetables, berries with some whipped cream and also nuts, seeds and avocados because these are healthy sources of carbohydrates.

And, try some good fats

Unlike what you're usually told, fats aren't all that bad. There are actually good and healthy kinds of fats that you need in your diet. Good fats provide you with energy and also help your body absorb nutrients easily plus they can also control or stabilize the body's cholesterol levels so you can live a healthy and well-balanced life. You can always start with mono-saturated fats, or those that are found mostly in oils and certain types of food. They decrease the risk of heart diseases and also control an insulin and blood sugar level which protects you from diabetes.

Then, you also can eat some poly-saturated fats, or fats found in oils and plant-based foods that can control cholesterol levels and protect you against heart diseases and certain types of cancer.

And of course, you shouldn't forget about Omega-3 Fatty Acids, which are found in tuna and most sea foods and are good because they keep the heart healthy and can reduce the risk of coronary heart disease, artery problems and irregular heartbeats. These fats also aid in weight loss.

Fat intake depends on your age, gender and lifestyle. Generally, adults and less active women should take 1,600 calories each day while less active men, active women and teenagers should take 2,200 calories or less and teenage boys, very active women and active men should take 2,500 calories or less each day. Doctors also recommend a 2,000 to 2,500 calorie diet or 44 to 78 grams of fat per day for everyone as a total of all kinds of healthy fats. Don't exceed the 2,500 mark because it might not be healthy for you and you may be an easy target of diseases.

If you're wondering where you could get healthy fats, here is a list of foods that are rich in healthy fats:

- **Seeds.** Seeds lower the amount of cholesterol in your body. Sunflower and Pumpkin Seeds are the best that you could try.

- **Peanut Butter.** This beloved sandwich spread is actually healthy for you because it is made up of mono-saturated fats. Choose finely ground ones instead of chunky/crispy ones with parts of nuts still in them. Now, you know that the classic Peanut Butter and Jelly Sandwich is actually good for you!

- **Omega 3 Fortified Foods.** Check labels of different food products and if you see that they are loaded with Omega 3, go for them. Oatmeal is one good example of this.

- **Olive Oil**. Use olive oil for cooking and you will be able to serve something healthy and good for the heart.

- **Nuts.** Nuts are also healthy sources of fats and what's great is that fats from nuts are good for the heart. Walnuts, Pecans and Hazelnuts provide you with ample amounts of nutrients. Make sure though that you don't eat them during every meal because it would be bad for your cholesterol levels. 1 ounce per meal per day would already be good. An ounce means around 35 peanuts, 24 almonds and 15 pecan halves. 18 cashews would also be good.

- **Kale, Spinach and Brussels sprouts.** These vegetables are good sources of fat and omega 3 fatty acids that keep the heart healthy and can protect you against various diseases, as mentioned in an earlier chapter. 2 to 3 cups of these greens each day would be beneficial for you so don't forget to add them to your shopping list.

- **Ground Flaxseed**. This contains enough soluble fiber that can rid your body of toxins and that will certainly protect you against various diseases. It's also the reason why flaxseed is all the rage these days when it comes to diet regimens. Use flaxseed for cereals or salads and you'll be alright.

- **Fish.** As mentioned earlier, omega 3 fatty acids are examples of healthy fats and you can get those from fish such as sardines, trout, tuna, herring, mackerel and salmon. Aside from being full of healthy fats, they also aid in keeping your brain sharp and smart. 2 servings of fatty fish each week is essential.

- **Eggs.** Eggs are not only a good source of fat, it's a good source of protein, too. An egg per day would definitely keep the doctor away.

- **Beans.** Kidney Beans, Navy Beans, Soybeans and Lentils boost your mood and strengthen the body, too.

- **Avocado.** What's good about avocado is that you can make different dishes and dips out of it. Make a guacamole, salsa or add it in your omelets or sandwiches and you'll certainly enjoy it. It prevents osteoarthritis and is definitely good for the heart, too. A medium avocado per serving can be good for you.

Compute carb and protein intake

You also should compute your carbohydrate and protein intake, and make sure that it falls under 1.2 grams per meal or around 30 grams each day. For this, compute the following:

1. Daily Carb Intake (grams)

2. Daily Protein Ratio (grams/lb.)

When you make use of proper portions, it'll be easier for you to follow the alkaline diet.

CHAPTER 7

How Acids Affect the Glycemic Index

The Glycemic Index or GI, is basically a guide that tells you how fast carbohydrates get into your bloodstream and turn into sugar, or glucose, which could affect the acidity in your body. There are free online calculators that would help you determine the said amounts but what this Chapter will tell you about is how you can manage your GI to make sure that it won't be so high. If you take in a lot of calories, as in more than 1,200 or 1,600, your GI might go higher than usual—so it's best that you take control of that. Basically, what's important is your body takes a long time to break down carbohydrates into sugar so your body won't be full of sugar and you won't suffer from various ailments. Here are some tips that will help you put your Glycemic Index under control:

1. Know that you can eat as many fruits and vegetables that you like. This is because fruits and vegetables are considered as "Water Foods", which means that they can do no harm to your blood sugar and won't contribute to worsening your situation. However, you have to avoid canned or preserved fruits or vegetables because there are preservatives used in them already and they'll only make your blood sugar levels higher.

2. Eat less-processed or unprocessed grains. No one's asking you to say goodbye to carbohydrates, but you have to make sure that you eat only the right kinds of them. This means that you should concentrate on wheat berries, brown rise, millet, and kernel dough instead of rice. Muesli or Granola Breakfast cereals are also fine.

3. Coal foods. Coal foods in particular won't contribute much to your GI because they are high in protein and fiber. Some of the best examples include beans, whole grains, seafood, lean meats, seeds, and nuts, as well as whole-wheat pasta.

4. Avoid fire foods. While coal foods are low in GI, fire foods are very high and that's exactly why you have to avoid them. Some examples include sweet chips, white pasta, white rice, white bread and most processed foods.

5. Stay away from starch. Starchy foods are not good for you because they contribute to your daily GI levels. This means that instead of eating those processed foods or chips for snacks, you should just eat fruits such as pears, papaya, berries, peaches, and apples because they're good for you and they'd add more water to your system.

6. Make sure that you chew your food well and that you eat slowly. When you're eating, you can take as much time as you want because if you chew your food well and if you're not eating in haste, it means that you will be able to avoid having high Glycemic Index and at the same time, you'd be able to make your metabolic rate go faster, too. When this happens, you get to burn fat quickly and so you also make sure that your health is in tip-top shape.

7. And, find alternatives to the usual foods that you eat. There are days when you seem to crave for foods that aren't really good for you and would just spike up your blood sugar levels. Well, what you can do is find an alternative and eat foods that are in the same category but would still keep your health in check. Check out the list below so you'll have a better idea of what this is about:

- Wild or brown rice instead of white rice.

- Whole wheat instead of regular pasta.

- Rolled or steel-cut oats instead of oatmeal.

- Raisin, oat, muesli, or granola instead of processed corn flakes or breakfast cereals.

- Mashed cauliflower, winter squash, yams, and sweet potatoes instead of mashed or fried white potatoes.

- Leafy greens or peas instead of corn.

- Bran flakes instead of cornflakes.

By following these tips, you can make sure that your Glycemic Index will be in check. In the next chapter, find out how you can still eat fats—even on an alkaline diet.

CHAPTER 8

Understanding Activity Levels and Energy Expenditures

You've also got to be mindful of energy expenditures and your activity levels. You see, when you remove acid in your system, your body becomes better—but not right away. This means that your body is still trying to adjust to the diet.

Now, you have to remember that it is important to workout, even just a bit, while you are on the diet so that you could help balance things out in your body—but you could not do this without knowing your activity levels first.

When it comes to Activity Levels, one thing that you have to understand is that what you eat should also be based on how much you move in a day. This way, you'd know how many calories your body is able to burn in just a day, and you'll also be able to take the right amount of fat, protein, and carbs. For this, you have the following to choose from:

- **Extremely Active**. It means you workout each day and that they are really intense (HIIT, *SoulCycle*, *PlanaForma,* etc.) You might be training twice a day, too.

- **Very Active.** This means that you partake in intense exercises at least 6 to 7 days a week.

- **Moderately Active**. This means you're physically tired each day, or have an active day job. It also means you work out at least 3 to 5 hours a week.

- **Lightly Active.** It means that you walk lightly each day, and that you endure 1 to 3 hours of light exercise.

- **Sedentary.** This means you do not really exercise—or only do a little of it, and that you don't partake in a lot of daily activities, too.

- This would help you understand how many calories your body is able to burn each day. For this, you need to compute:

- **Basal Metabolic Rate (BMR).** This is the minimal energy expenditure rate or the amount of time used by the body when it's producing energy at rest. This involves your age, weight, and gender.

- **Thermic Effect of Food**. This is the heat production that happens in the body, courtesy of the brown adipose tissue that is activated each time you consume a meal. You should measure this 1 to 5 hours after eating—just input whatever you ate on your last meal.

Once you get to compute your energy expenditure, that's when you can decide on which alkaline foods would work well for you, and the kind of workouts that are actually perfect for you.

CHAPTER 9

Specifics of Alkaline Cooking

Trying a new diet really isn't just about knowing the right kinds of food to eat, but also knowing the right ways to cook or prepare them, or to make substitutes when the situation calls for it.

Simple Cooking Tips

- You can't have Pasta, but you can always make your own pasta by using spaghetti squash, instead.

- You can make use of your extra dinner as lunch for the following day.

- You can make one huge salad at the start of the week, and then make use of some of the ingredients for the rest of the week. Basically, you can mix and match ingredients—as long as you keep them fresh in the fridge!

- You can also cook meat in bulk.

- The adjustment period may take time. That's a given. But that doesn't mean that you have to give up right away. Remember that every good thing actually takes time, so just hang in there.

- Omelets always work for breakfast.

- Never use same sifters from various flours. Again, doing so would prevent cross-contamination from happening.

- Never prepare gluten and Alkaline foods on the same surface.

- Never ever forget to read labels. These would help you understand whether what you're having—or adding to your meals—is Alkaline, or not.

- Make homemade broth and make sure to consume it. It would make your immune system stronger, and you can always use the broth as base for your soups and stews, too.

- It would be best to plan your meals for the rest of the week. It would also be best if you don't try to hasten preparation time, too.

- It would be best to have separate utensils meant only for cooking Alkaline dishes and another set of utensils only for your Non-Gluten Free meals. This way, cross contamination could be avoided.

- If you're having a party, or eating with people who have Celiac Disease, or Gluten allergies, it would be best to make sure that they do not share the same dips. Also, do not let crumbs go into the dips, as well.

- Don't use the same toasters for various kinds of breads.

- Don't cook and eat without moving. You have to aid the Alkaline Diet with some movement AKA exercise. Even simple brisk walking would do.

Alkaline foods should never be deep-fried. If you're eating out, make sure to ask the restaurant staff about whether breaded and unbreaded products have been cooked in the same surface or not.

- Stick with it for at least 30 days. It's said that the Alkaline Diet would work best if you'd learn how to stick with it for at least a month. At this rate, your body would learn how to adjust to it, and would consider it a regular part of your life!

Use alkaline-friendly flours

These are:

- **Arrowroot Flour.** This is one of the best thickeners you can get out there, and is actually tasteless when cooked.

- **Buckwheat Flour.** While it has wheat in its name, you can relax because it's not actually wheat. It's from the rhubarb family, and would give your dishes a nutty flavor.

- **Brown Rice Flour.** This is bran-milled flour that has an earthy flavor and is best for making gnocchi.

- **White Rice Flour.** This may be a bit bland, but gives your recipes a light and easy to eat texture.

- **Rice Flour.** This one has delicate texture when cooked and is great for making sponge cakes and noodles.

- **Tapioca Flour.** This is pretty chewy and is perfect for patties and casseroles.

- **Soya Flour.** Made from soybeans, this one has quite a nutty taste and is said to be one of the best alternatives to flour.

- **Quinoa Flour.** Quinoa is related to spinach and has been around for over 5,000 years. It works best for desserts, such as pastries and cakes.

Use alkaline substitutes

Make sure that the way you cook won't be detrimental to your health by learning how to make use of Alkaline Substitutes. For these, you can try the following:

Trail Mix. Trail Mixes could be fun with the help of alkaline chips, candies, dried fruits, raisins, and peanuts. Don't buy date trail mixes as they're usually rolled in non-gluten free oat flours.

Thickeners. For thickeners, you can use tapioca starch or arrowroot flour. Dry pudding could work, too.

Soy and Teriyaki Sauce. You can mostly use Liquid Aminos, which you can usually find at health stores. You could also make use of most Asian Sauces, or choose to make your own teriyaki sauce by mixing soy sauce substitute with equal parts of wine and sugar, too.

Pie Crust. Basically, you could just turn crusted recipes into non-crusted ones. Say, quiche without the crust or something. However, if you're trying to make pastry, it would be best to just crush alkaline cereals or cookies and press them onto a greased pie pan. Bake the way you would a regular pie and you're all set!

Hot Breakfast/Oatmeal. You can mostly use corn grits. Fry them, and add sugar, cinnamon, or butter. Quinoa and Amaranth cereals could work, too.

Granola. You can make your own Alkaline Granola by tossing spices, seasoning, some oil, vanilla, honey, alkaline cereal, seeds, and nuts altogether. Bake at 300 degrees for around an hour and add dried fruits shortly before serving.

Flour. Alkaline flours, and Cornstarch could work. Amaranth is often the number 1 choice, but feel free to choose whatever you want.

Flour and Bun Tortillas. You should make use of rice wraps, available in most Thai/Asian stores. You can also use corn tortillas, alkaline bread, and lettuce. You can also use *Nori* for stuffing—just like you would with sushi.

Croutons. For croutons, you can make use fo Alkaline bread mixed with Parmesan cheese.

Breading and Coatings. Make use of alkaline breadcrumbs, crushed potato chips, corn flour, or corn meal for your coating needs.

Binders. Make use of guar gum, xanthan gum, or gelatin.

CHAPTER 10

Diseases That Could Be Prevented—or Alleviated—by the Alkaline Diet

Cancer

Research has it that with the help of catechins, a form of antioxidant found in Alkaline Foods, free radicals are sought and destroyed on the spot. This only means that when free radicals are destroyed, the body gets to be saved from most diseases—as well as Cancer.

A study done in *McGill University* shows that Alkaline Foods's antioxidants are able to shrink tumors that are mostly found in mice. Lung Cancer risk is also lessened by up to 18%, also due to Alkaline Foods.

Now, when one has already suffered from the past, relapse could be prevented with the help of alkaline foods in the sense that an increase of green alkaline foods intake prevents cancer cells from forming, mostly by destroying mitochondria—the cell that's responsible for creating cancer cells in the body.

Pancreatic, colorectal, and prostate cancer are likewise prevented.

Heart Diseases

Studies show that green alkaline foods lower LDL or bad cholesterol by up to 35%. When this happens, the heart will be protected and strokes could be prevented.

More so, alkaline foods could also prevent fat buildup. Usually, people with heavier weights are those who are susceptible to heart diseases because fat is already adamant in their bloodstream. When alkaline foods are part of one's regular diet, the more it protects the body from elements that may damage the heart.

One Japanese case study has shown that 4 out of 5 men who have added alkaline foods to their diet have shown life longevity—without any heart problems!

Arthritis

Arthritis happens because of inflammation. If you've been reading this book properly, you'd know that there are actually various kinds of alkaline foods that help prevent inflammation, especially when added with other ingredients.

The thing is, compounds found in alkaline foods reverses the effects of responses that are usually associated with arthritis, diabetes, and other inflammatory problems.

The breakdown of cartilage walls is also prevented, making sure that arthritis patients are safe from further damage. You see, alkaline foods help keep a person's condition stable, instead of letting it worsen— and that's one of the best things that it can do.

Diabetes

Another amazing thing about Alkaline Foods is that it could help normalize blood sugar levels—and doing so would prevent another one of the most debilitating diseases out there—diabetes.

This happens because alkaline foods regulate the body's glucose levels—and in turn, turn said glucose to energy. Now, when this happens, one would be stronger, and would also be able to use the energy for more important things, instead of letting a disease consume the body.

Cell and Tissue Damage

As said earlier, alkaline foods are full of antioxidants that slow the process of aging down, and that also wards diseases off. Alkaline foods also repair damaged cells, and makes sure that free radicals do not get to them. More so, these antioxidants also prevent the growth of cancer cells, as well as high cholesterol levels, and also dilate blood vessels to improve energy and elasticity in the body. This also prevents clogging of the blood, and makes sure there's proper antioxidant concentration in the body.

Autoimmune Diseases

As often reiterated in this book, you can expect that with the help of alkaline foods, the aging process is slowed down—so you could still look and stay healthy even while you're growing older. Studies done have shown a lot of promise when it comes to alkaline food's effects on the immune system—which definitely is a good thing.

Remember, alkaline food is something that you could add in your daily diet. Don't try to let all the myths about it fool you—it's definitely amazing and safe!

CHAPTER 11

FAQs

If you're having doubts as to the credibility and benefits of this diet, then here are some commonly asked questions about it—answered for your convenience!

Q: Can alkaline foods also prevent Alzheimer's Disease?

A: According to a couple of studies done over the years, especially those performed by the *University of Newcastle*, Alkaline Foods actually improves memory, and when one's memory is good, Alzheimer's Disease could be prevented in the long run.

This is because alkaline foods affect the cholinergic system of the brain, which, when damaged, contributes to the risk of getting Alzheimer's in the future. Alkaline foods hydrolyze the enzymes that could destroy the said system, and therefore get to protect the brain from further damage.

Also, studies have shown that alkaline food contains the same elements as pharmaceutical products do—minus the side effects, and while working for a long period of time. This means that the effects will not only be prevalent today, but as long as one has alkaline foods in his diet.

Q: Is it true that alkaline foods are good for healthy aging?

A: Yes, absolutely.

Since alkaline foods restore the skin's elasticity due to its antioxidant content, healthy aging is promoted. Take for example those in countries that naturally drink alkaline foods (i.e., Japan)—you can see that they age gracefully, compared to those who just drink it occasionally, and whose diets are mostly made up of preservatives.

Research also has it that those who drink alkaline foods live longer—without having to worry about diseases that old age could bring.

Q: Can the quality of water affect the quality of alkaline foods?

A: Yes, it could.

You know, alkaline foods actually taste better when polyphenols and caffeine meet each other, and work together—and this only happens when you get to brew alkaline foods properly, and not in overcooked or over boiled water.

Overcooked water dampens the taste of the alkaline foods. When it's no longer palatable, you may feel like you shouldn't add it in your diet anymore—and that's what you have to prevent from happening.

Q: Can alkaline foods prevent stroke?

A: When eaten regularly, yes, there is a chance.

This is because alkaline foods contain polyphenols and antioxidants that the body easily absorbs to protect itself from free radicals that may bring forth stroke and cancer. While doing so, it also clears the digestive tract, and could also protect one from most degenerative diseases, too.

Q: Are alkaline foods bad for pregnant women?

A: First and foremost, this is just a myth.

Studies show that consuming alkaline foods has no effects to either the pregnant and lactating mother, or to her child, whether through growth retention, or miscarriages. There are also no effects of alkaline foods caffeine on child development and mental processes.

However, when one already has an aversion to alkaline foods, and often suffers from indigestion when consuming caffeine, it's best to consult the doctor first before drinking alkaline foods. It's also best to eat a healthy diet and exercise regularly even when one is pregnant, so that birth will be easy, and so the woman would be able to maintain good health while taking care of her child, as well.

A pregnant woman could drink up to 3 to 4 cups of alkaline foods each day, but has to refrain from coffee as it may bring forth palpitations.

Q: Are alkaline foods really good for my immune system?

A: Yes, especially when you take it regularly. This is because it boosts the body's capability to bring infection down, and could also track germs better—so the immune system could drive them away from the body.

Q: It's said that alkaline food blocks iron absorption. Is this true?

A: Absolutely not.

Dietary iron has two forms, which are non-heme iron (plant iron), and heme iron (animal iron). When you consume alkaline foods, your body still gets to absorb at least 15 to 35% of heme, and 25% of non-heme iron—which means you'd get the amazing dietary benefits that they bring.

It's also easy to absorb polyphenols and ascorbic acid with the help of alkaline foods, as well.

Q: What makes the Flat Alkaline Foods Belly Diet healthy? What are the nutrients that one could get from alkaline foods?

A: As there are various kinds of alkaline food, you can expect that nutritional content varies, too. But mostly, you can expect that you'll get the following:

- **Sodium**. Sodium prevents hypertension.

- **Protein**. Protein is one of the most important nutrients that the body needs to function well. You can get at least 2% or more of it from one cup of alkaline foods.

- **Potassium**. Potassium helps cells do their job properly. Alkaline foods contain a lot of potassium.

- **Magnesium**. Magnesium is essential for the strength and growth of the human body, and could also prevent tissue breakage.

- **Lipids.** Lipids are good kinds of fat that are mostly mixed with protein and could help hair become stronger.

- **Fluorine.** Fluorine helps make teeth stronger.

- **Carbohydrates.** Alkaline foods contain around 4 to 5% of carbohydrates—so you could omit rice and other grains from your diet.

- **Calcium and Phosphorous.** These are both needed for bones to grow strong. Teeth could benefit from them, too.

Also, you could expect that with the help of alkaline foods, you will get to fill your dietary needs by getting:

6% Vitamin B6

25% Vitamin B2

9% Vitamin B1

10% Zinc

16% Calcium

Around 50% of flavonoids and anti-oxidants.

In short, if you want to live a healthy life, you definitely should add alkaline foods in your diet.

CHAPTER 12

Important Tips to Keep in Mind

Finally, here are important alkaline diet tips that you definitely shouldn't forget!

- Balance your protein and carb intake. Protein is one of the best macronutrients in life but the problem is that sometimes, people tend to overeat protein—mostly because they have not managed their macros. When you eat more protein than you need, what happens is that the body does not get in the state of Ketosis—which might make it hard for you to get through each day. Now, what you can do here is make sure that you aim for just 1.5 to 2.0 grams of protein per kilogram of bodyweight each day. This way, gluconeogenesis—or the process of transforming glucose into energy—could happen. Aside from computing your macros and aiming for at least 50 grams of carbs per day, you also should do a carbohydrate sweep. In short, you have to dispose of carbohydrates that are taking space in your cupboards or fridge. These include the following: fruit juice, fruit juice concentrates, tapioca syrup, galactose, lactose, fructose, barley malt, maltose, agave nectar, honey, brown sugar syrup, panela, caramel, date sugar, coconut sugar, white sugar, sucrose, corn sweetener, corn syrup, cane juice, cane sugar, brown sugar, and turbinado sugar. You also should take away grains and grain products, such as pretzels, pies, tortillas, crackers, cold cereals, waffles, and white bread. Canned soups and starchy vegetables should not be in your grocery list, too.

- Make sure not to drink too much alcohol as this increases blood pressure. You can drink coffee but make sure to keep it under control.

- Tuna, herring, and salmon are the best kinds of fish out there, when fiber content is concerned.

- If you really love sweets, make sure to choose those that are low-fat or fat-free such as jelly beans, fruit ices, sorbets, or graham crackers. Make sure to check nutritional labels for added sugar. Avoid products with added sugar as much as possible.

- Fat-free or low-fat yogurt will help you curb those dairy cravings. Yogurt's healthy and can be considered as a sweet treat, too. It's best added with fruits, which you'll also be learning about later.

- Grains can be eaten for most of the day because they are rich in fiber and low in fat. Make sure to look for those that are labeled "100 percent whole wheat" or "100 percent whole grain".

- Always make sure that you skin meat, poultry and fish and that you bake instead of frying.

- You can use both fresh and frozen vegetables—not just as side dishes, but as main meals. You'll find some recipes in the next chapters that makes use of vegetables.

- If you're lactose-intolerant, make sure that you choose only lactose-free products.

- As much as possible, don't use too much salt in your recipes and make sure to buy foods that are labeled as "very low sodium", "sodium free", or "no salt added".

- Don't eat regular kinds of cheese too much as they are loaded with sodium.

- Fat-free or low-fat yogurt will help you curb those dairy cravings. Yogurt's healthy and can be considered as a sweet treat, too. It's best added with fruits, which you'll also be learning about later.

- And, be patient! Some people forget that the Alkaline Diet—as well as other diet plans—would not work like magic. If it did, it means it's probably not a real diet—and that's not what you'd want to experience. Take note that it would take days for the body to adapt to this new diet because it's probably not used to a high-fat diet. If you feel a bit sick, it means you're experiencing the low-carb flu—and that's pretty normal for people who are switching to the Alkaline Diet. This would last for around 3 to 4 days, and in a matter of weeks, your body would fully be able to adjust to the Alkaline Diet. Remember that this is not something you should be worried about, and focus on doing what the diet asks you to do.

Keep these tips in mind and soon enough, you'd be able to live a healthy life—one that's free of acid, and is definitely enjoyable, thanks to the alkaline diet.

For a comprehensive list of foods in this diet, refer to the next chapter.

CHAPTER 13

A Complete List of Alkalizing and Acidifying Foods

Here is a complete food guide to help you reorganize your meals so you can be on your way to alkalizing your body and gaining better health.

Alkalinity Ranking

The following ranks the different alkaline-inducing foods according to how effective they are in promoting alkalinity.

Extremely Alkaline Forming Foods are those that leave residue with pH 8.5 to 9.0. Extremely Acid Forming Foods are those that leave residue with pH 5.0 to 5.5. These are sample foods that give the specific pH, based on the ash or residue they produce in the body after they are burned or metabolized:

Extremely Alkaline Foods

At pH 9

- Lemons are extremely alkaline.

- Watermelon is a wonderful fruit to include in a yearly fast. Eat whole watermelon for a number of days (about 2-3 days). Chew the watermelon pips well and eat. This is a super alkalizing food to include in the alkaline diet.

At pH 8.5

- Agar agar, which is a healthier alternative to gelatin

- Asparagus, which is a potent reducer of acidity in the body. It helps detoxify the body. Asparagus will temporarily cause your urine to become more acidic as it promotes the removal of excess acid in your body.

- Fruit juices, those with natural sugars that promote alkalinity. Added sugars to fruit juices will make them acid-forming

- Vegetable juices, but this will depend on the type of vegetable that is included and the sweetness of the vegetable juice

- Cayenne

- Cantaloupe *also on p.85 as moderately alkaline*

- Dried figs and dates

- Kudzu root

- Endive

- Kiwifruit

- Karengo

- Mango

- Limes

- Passion fruit

- Melons

- Papaya

- Umeboshi plum

- Raisins

- Sweet seedless grapes

- Sweet Pears

- Pineapple

- Parsley

- Watercress

- Kelp

- Seaweeds

Highly Alkaline Forming Foods

- Baking soda

- Sea salt

- Mineral water

- Pumpkin seed

- Lentils

- Seaweed

- Taro root

- Lotus root

- Persimmon

- Tangerine

- Pineapple

Moderately Alkaline (foods with residue pH ranging from 7.5 to 8.0)

At pH 8.0

- Sea salt (vegetable), the vegetable component is what raises the alkalinity of the body

- Garlic, which is great to add to foods with pH 5 to turn into a more alkaline pH

- Sweet Apples

- Apricots

- Arrowroot

- Ripe bananas

- Avocados

- Guavas

- Pears (less sweet)

- Berries

- Grapes (less sweet)

- Gooseberry

- Currants

- Grapefruit

- Sweet peaches

- Nectarine

- Carrots

- Fresh dates & figs

- Alfalfa sprouts

- Lettuce (leafy green)

- Celery

- Herbs (leafy green)

- Peas (fresh sweet)

- Pumpkin (sweet)

- Persimmon

- Spinach

At pH 7.5

- Apple cider vinegar – Its raw unpasteurized version aids in digestion, increasing the amounts of HCl in the stomach to promote better digestion of food. To use, mix 1 tablespoon of apple cider vinegar with water and honey. Take before meals.

- Squash - The winter squash variety has a pH value of 7.5 while the butternut and sweeter squash varieties rate at pH 8.0

- Sour apples

- Bamboo shoots

- Fresh green Beans

- Beets

- Bell Pepper

- Broccoli

- Cauliflower

- Cabbage

- Carob

- Fresh Ginger

- Sour grapes

- Oranges

- Not so sweet peaches

- Raspberry

- Strawberry

- Kohlrabi

- Kale

- Pale green lettuce

- Peas (less sweet)

- Potatoes with the skin on

- Pumpkin (less sweet)

- Sapote

- Fresh sweet corn

- Tamari

- Daikon

- Parsnip

- Turnip

Other Moderately Alkaline Foods

- Apples (sweet apples more moderately alkaline than sour variety)

- Lettuce (leafy green more moderately alkaline than pale green variety)

- Grapes (less sweet more moderately alkaline than sour varieties)

- Peaches (sweet variety more moderately alkaline than less sweet fruit)

- Peas (fresh and sweet more moderately alkaline than the less sweet variety)

- Pumpkin (sweet pumpkin more moderately alkaline than less sweet one)

- Citrus

- Currants

- Cantaloupe *on p. 80 as extremely alkaline which is it?*

- Loganberry

- Honeydew

- Dewberry

- Parsley

- Spices

- Arugula

- Mustard green

- Endive

- Asparagus

- Sea salt

- Beans (fresh, green)

- Pepper

- Olive

- Squash

- Kombucha

- Soy sauce

- Unsulfured molasses

- Chestnuts

- Cashews

Slightly Alkaline to Neutral pH 7.0

At pH 7.0

- Almonds, soak the unblanched whole nuts for 12 hours, then peel the skin off before eating.

- Ripe olives, either sundried or tree ripened. Other varieties have pH 6.0.

- Pickles, made with apple cider vinegar and sea salt

- Essene bread, more alkaline if made with sprouted grains. As the grains are chewed well, they become more alkaline.

- Barley-Malt (sweetener-Bronner)

- Millet

- Quinoa

- Brown Rice Syrup

- Vinegar from sweet brown rice

- Spices, various types range from pH 7.0 to 8.0

- Homemade mayonnaise

- Olive oil

- Sea salt

- Artichokes (Jerusalem)

- Artichoke (globe)

- Brussel sprouts

- Cherries

- Fresh coconut

- Cucumbers

- Raw honey

- Leeks

- Eggplant

- Onions

- Mushrooms

- Okra

- Horseradish

- Radish

- Taro

- Amaranth

- Tomatoes

- Water Chestnut

- Dry roasted chestnuts

- Whole sesame seeds

- Raw goat's milk and whey

- Egg yolks (soft cooked)

- Rhubarb

- Dry soy beans

- Soy milk

- Soy cheese

- Sprouted grains

- Tofu

- Tempeh

- Miso

- Yeast (nutritional flakes)

Other Slightly Alkaline foods

- Tomatoes (sweet tomatoes are slightly more alkaline than the less sweet version)
- Whole Sesame seeds

Low Alkaline Forming Foods

- Most herbs (non-leafy)
- Mu tea
- Green tea
- Sake
- Rice syrup
- Quail eggs
- Ginseng
- Primrose oil
- Cod liver oil
- Sesame seed
- Collard green
- Sprouts
- Rutabaga
- Cherry
- Blackberry
- Papaya

Very Low Alkaline Forming Foods

- Ginger tea
- Grain coffee
- Umeboshi vinegar
- Duck eggs
- Ghee
- Currant
- Oats
- Japonica rice
- Quinoa
- Wild rice
- Flax oil
- Avocado oil
- Coconut oil
- Most seeds
- Cilantro
- Chive
- Turnip greens

Neutral pH

- Fresh unsalted butter

- Fresh and raw cream

- Margarine – Avoid heating it because heat hardens the fat contents and make them difficult to digest

- Raw cow's milk

- Oils, except olive oil

- Whey from cow's milk

- Plain yogurt

Slightly acidic to Neutral pH

At slightly below pH 7.0

- Bran

- Barley

- Rye (grain)

- Cereals, unrefined and served with honey-fruit-maple syrup

- Cornmeal

- Barley malt syrup

- Unprocessed maple syrup

- Unsulfured organic molasses

- Pasteurized Honey

- Fructose

- Macadamias
- Brazil nuts
- Pistachios
- Walnuts
- Cashews
- Pecans
- Homogenized milk
- Homogenized goats' milk
- Most processed dairy products
- Egg whites
- Mustard
- Nutmeg
- Popcorn & plain butter
- Rye bread made from organic sprouted grains
- Rice or wheat crackers (unrefined)
- Seeds (pumpkin & sunflower)
- Blueberries
- Cranberries
- Salted butter
- Crackers from unrefined rye grains

- Cheeses (mild & crumbly)

- Lentils

- Dried beans (mung, adzuki, pinto, kidney, garbanzo), sprouted dried beans become more alkaline, at pH 7.0

- Dry coconut

- Pickled olives

- Plums and prunes, contain quinic and benzoic acids, which are acid-forming compounds in the body

- Spelt

Moderately acidic foods

At pH 6.5

- Green bananas

- Egg whole (hard boiled)

- Sharp cheeses

- Peanuts

- Potatoes without skins

- Popcorn (with salt & butter)

- Buckwheat

- Basmati rice

- Brown rice

- Oats

- Tapioca
- Whole grain Pasta
- Wholegrain & honey pastry
- Wheat bread made from sprouted organic grains
- Corn & rice breads
- Ketchup
- Mayonnaise
- Commercial soy sauce

At pH 6.0

- Cigarette tobacco (rolled on your own)
- Cream of Wheat (unrefined)
- Sweetened Yogurt
- Fruit juices with sugar
- Fish
- Shellfish
- Sulfured molasses
- Processed maple syrup
- Commercial pickles
- Refined cereals such as Weetbix, corn flakes
- Breads made from refined corn, oats, rice & rye

- Whole wheat foods. Unrefined wheat ad wheat products are more alkaline

- Wheat germ

- Wine

Other Moderately Acidic Foods

- Blueberries

- Plums

- Prunes

- Cranberries

- Barley (rye)

- Bran

- Oats (rye, organic)

- Crackers (unrefined rye, rice and wheat)

- Cereals (unrefined)

- Butter (regular)

- Cheeses

- Egg whites

- Fructose

- Honey (pasteurized)

- Mustard

- Maple syrup (unprocessed)

- Molasses (unsulfured and organic)

- Most nuts

- Seeds (pumpkin, sunflower)Dry coconut

- Olives (pickled)

- Soy sauce

- Bear

- Casein

- Cottage cheese

- Milk protein

- Nutmeg

- Squid

- Mussels

- Maize

- Corn

- Barley groats

- Oat bran

- Rye

- Chestnut oil

- Palm kernel oil

- Lard

- Pecans
- Pistachio seeds
- Green peas
- Snow peas
- Garbanzo beans
- Other legumes
- Pomegranate

Very Low Acid Forming Foods

- Curry
- koma coffee
- Honey
- Goat/sheep cheese
- Chicken
- Gelatin
- Organs
- Venison
- Wild duck
- Triticale
- Millet
- Kasha

- Amaranth
- Brown rice
- Pumpkin seed oil
- Grape seed oil
- Sunflower oil
- Pine nuts
- Canola oil
- Spinach
- Fava beans
- Black-eyed peas
- String beans
- Wax beans
- Zucchini
- Chutney
- Rhubarb
- Dry fruit

Low Acid Forming Foods

- Vanilla
- Balsamic vinegar
- Black tea

- Cow milk
- Goat milk
- Aged cheese
- Game meat
- Boar
- Mutton
- Elk
- Mollusks
- Shell fish
- Turkey
- Goose
- Wheat
- Buckwheat
- Spelt
- Kamut
- Teff
- Farina
- White rice
- Semolina
- Almond oil

- Safflower oil

- Sesame oil

- Seitan

- Tapioca

- Pinto beans

- Navy beans

- White beans

- Red beans

- Lima beans

- Aduki beans

- Chard

Extremely acidic foods

At pH 5.5

- Beef

- Goat

- Lamb

- Pork

- Carbonated soft drinks & fizzy drinks

- Flour (white, wheat), if bleached, these types of flour have no nutritional value.

- Pastries & cakes from white flour

- White or refined sugar has no nutritional value. In fact, it is considered as poison.

- Cigarettes (tailor made)

- Drugs

- Beer, good quality and well brewed beer has pH reaching up to 5.5. Beer that's fast brewed has more acid, dropping down to pH 5.0.

- Brown sugar

- Chicken

- Deer

- Chocolate

- Coffee, organic and fresh ground has pH reaching to 5.5

- Custard with white sugar

- Jams

- Jellies

- Liquor, cheaper liquor bands have very low pH, dropping to as low as pH 5.0

- White pasta

- Rabbit

- Semolina

- Table salt refined and iodized

- Tea black

- Turkey
- Wheat bread
- White rice
- White vinegar (processed).

At pH 5.0

- Artificial sweeteners

Extremely Acidic

- Artificial sweeteners
- Cigarettes and tobacco
- Liquor
- Carbonated soft drinks
- Soft drinks, especially the cola type (*Surprising fact*: Neutralizing just 1 glass of cola, which has a pH of 2.5, would require drinking 32 glasses of alkaline water, which has a pH of 10)
- Fruit juices with sugar
- Beer
- Coffee
- Chocolate
- Beef
- Lamb

- Deer
- Fish
- Pork
- Lobster
- Pheasant
- Seafood
- Poultry
- Fried foods
- Drugs
- Most breads
- Flour (white, wheat)
- White bread
- Pastries and cakes from white flour
- Whole wheat foods
- Pasta (white)
- Brown sugar
- Cream of wheat (unrefined)
- Cereals (refined)
- Yogurt (sweetened)
- Pudding
- Custard (with white sugar)

- Molasses (sulfured)

- Maple syrup (processed)

- Jellies

- Jams

- Pickles (commercial)

- White vinegar (processed)

- Table salt (refined and iodized)

- Sugar (white)

- Tea (black)

- Wine

- Tabletop sweeteners like (NutraSweet, Sweet 'N Low, Aspartame, Equal or Spoonful)

- Hops

- Malt

- Barley

- Sugar

- Cocoa

- White (acetic acid) vinegar

- Processed cheese

- Ice cream

- Cottonseed oil

- Hazelnuts

- Walnuts

- Brazil nuts

- Soybean

Alkaline activity: It's not just food that produces alkalinity or acidity in the body. In the alkaline diet, even activities are also important. Alkaline activities are also emphasized to improve the pH balance in the body, aside from making heathier food choices.

Alkaline promoting activities include:

- Prayer

- Meditation

- Love

- Kindness

- Peace

Acidic activities: There are also activities that promote the formation of more acid in the body. Limit these activities to prevent yourself from suffering from more health problems related to too much acid in the body. Acid promoting activities include:

- Stress

- Anger

- Overwork

- Jealousy

- Fear

Conclusion

Thank you again for purchasing this book!

I hope this book was able to help you to understand and ultimately follow the alkaline diet. The body has its own homeostatic processes to keep everything in balance, but certain things can make it harder for the body to heal and balance itself. By going on an alkaline diet, the body is aided in maintaining its balance and reducing risks for health problems.

The next step is to start making changes. Add more alkaline foods and limit eating acid-forming foods.

Finally, if you enjoyed this book, please take the time to share your thoughts and post a review on Amazon. I want to reach as many people as I can with this book, and more reviews will help me accomplish that. It'd be greatly appreciated!

Thank you and good luck!

CPSIA information can be obtained
at www.ICGtesting.com
Printed in the USA
FSOW03n2057210517
34518FS